PRESENTED TO

_____

FROM

_____

Dedicated to everyone whose life

has been touched by cancer,

and played a role

in their care and recovery.

CHRISTINE CLIFFORD, CSP

How Can
I Help?

Giving and Receiving
Kindness & Care
When You or Someone You Love
Has Cancer

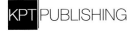KPT PUBLISHING

When we hear or learn that someone we care about has cancer, often we don't know what to say or do. Perhaps we end up saying nothing for fear of saying the "wrong" thing. Or we do reach out but send a "silent gesture" of support—a card, flowers, or perhaps an email. Our silence can make the cancer patient feel even more alone.

What can we do?

This little book was designed to give you some unique ideas that I have tried with wonderful results to help make the life of a cancer patient just a little bit easier; a little less stressful; and perhaps even a little more fun.

Thank you for being a caregiver, a friend, or a beloved family member. Anyone reading this book who has taken a step to provide support is among the true Guardian Angels of our world.

"There's an elephant in the room.

We all know it is there.

We are thinking about the elephant

As we talk together.

It is constantly on our minds.

For, you see, it is a very big elephant.

It has hurt us all.

About the elephant in the room."

❧

TERRY KETTERING

DID YOU
HEAR
the news?

There is a rollercoaster of emotions that touch us all when we learn a loved one or friend has cancer. It is human nature to back away from unpleasant situations; however, it is often in this initial phase of shock that cancer patients need the most help.

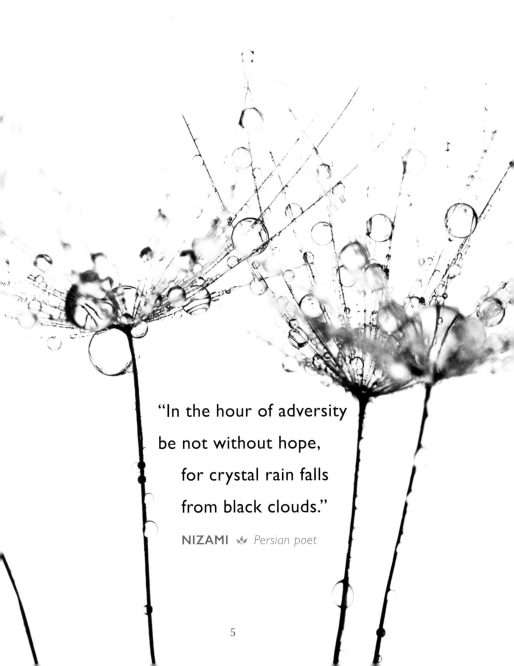

"In the hour of adversity
be not without hope,
for crystal rain falls
from black clouds."

NIZAMI ❧ *Persian poet*

We probably remember the day we learned someone we love or care for was diagnosed with cancer. The word "cancer" can spread through cell phones and email like wildfire, causing the patient to feel like a fish in a fishbowl. During this critical time, use judgement as a family member or friend wisely, calling only the closest friends and family members of the patient— with their permission. Wait until you have accurate facts and information to share before making calls. Give the patient a few days to get acclimated to the news before you ask to help. At this point, the newly diagnosed patient is simply trying to overcome the shock of hearing those words: "I'm so sorry. You have cancer."

Call your closest companion and ask them to come over to comfort you. Share the news of your diagnosis and allow yourselves to cry and grieve. Then together decide who else you need to call right away, and who should make the calls. Try to focus on just those people in your inner circle who you can trust and will maintain your privacy.

BOOKS
and the
INTERNET
Your New "Best Friend"

After the initial shock and tears, most cancer patients want to learn as much as possible about their disease. It is at this point in the journey that friends and family can begin contributing knowledge, personal experiences, and research to help the patient grasp their illness.

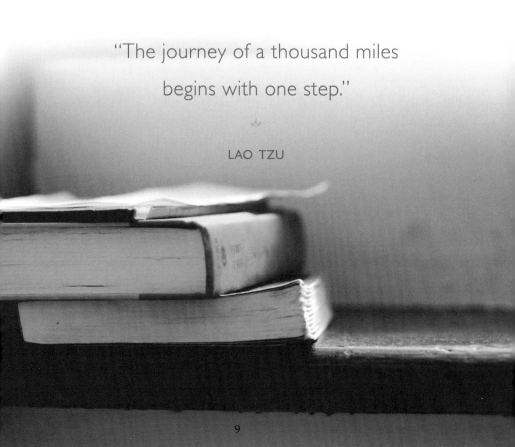

"The journey of a thousand miles

begins with one step."

LAO TZU

eceiving a diagnosis of cancer is the most stressful time in someone's life, and most people don't
know where to go or who to turn to. Visit your local
library or bookstore and get one or two general books
on cancer that will help explain the types of doctors
your friend or loved one needs to see; different terms
regarding treatments and procedures; and facts relating
to their specific type of cancer. Offer to help make calls
to get physician referrals, and volunteer to call to make
appointments. Drive the patient to consultations and be
available to help "take notes." Your friend or loved one
will be grateful for the support and glad someone else
has a second "pair of ears."

Let a friend or loved one help you navigate the new and often frightening world of doctors, hospitals, and clinics by allowing them to make some phone calls and drive you to your appointments. By asking them to record the doctor's comments, you will be grateful to have the notes to refer back to when you get home and begin to sort things out.

The
JOURNEY
BEGINS
at the
Hospital

These days most patients in the hospital for cancer surgery are out before they knew what hit them! Visitors, calls, and flowers are always welcomed. Support for the families of cancer patients is more important now than ever.

"They might not need me,

but they might,

I'll let my head be just in sight;

A smile as small as mine might be

Precisely their necessity."

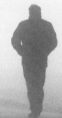

EMILY DICKINSON

acing surgery for cancer treatment can be as frightening for the caregiver of a cancer patient as it is for patients themselves. Often the caregiver feels isolated, confused, and unsure of what he/she can do in the situation. Organize a "comfort" party in the lobby area of the hospital on the day of the surgery. Invite family, friends, employers, and neighbors to drop by and offer their support. Encourage people to bring food and beverages along with a guest book that can be signed with words of encouragement from the attendees. Then the caregiver can present it to the cancer patient when he/she comes out of surgery and is recovering in their room. Both the patient and the caregiver will feel the love and support, and won't feel quite so alone in the experience.

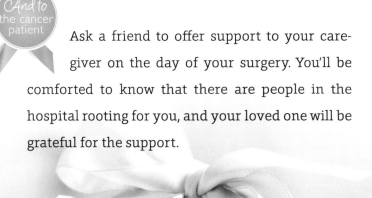

Ask a friend to offer support to your care-giver on the day of your surgery. You'll be comforted to know that there are people in the hospital rooting for you, and your loved one will be grateful for the support.

COMING HOME

This is the prime time to connect with a cancer patient to let them know that they are in your thoughts and prayers, and that you are thinking of them. "Silent gestures" of friendship (cards, hand-written notes, flowers, etc.) will let the patient know that you've heard about their situation and are there to support them.

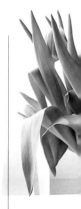

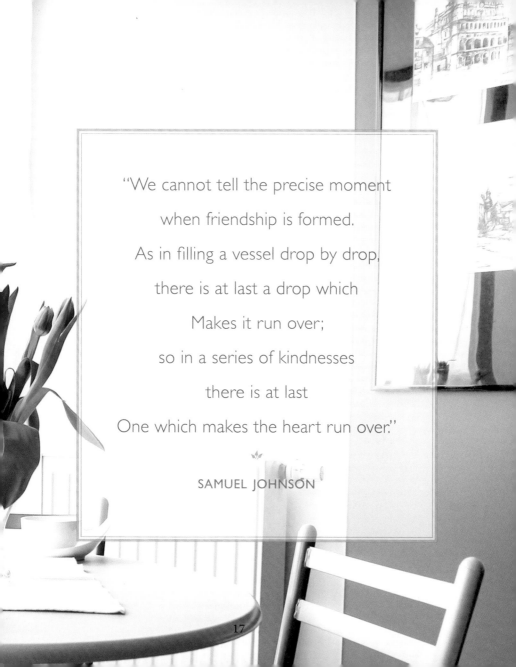

"We cannot tell the precise moment

when friendship is formed.

As in filling a vessel drop by drop,

there is at last a drop which

Makes it run over;

so in a series of kindnesses

there is at last

One which makes the heart run over."

SAMUEL JOHNSON

*E*ven a person with the best and brightest attitude can feel "out of sorts" from the stress and anxiety from surgery. Send a gift certificate for a body massage, facial, scalp massage, manicure, or pedicure to help soothe the soul and brighten spirits. Even a simple certificate for a "shampoo and blow-dry" can mean the world to someone coming out of surgery with not a lot of energy. You will have helped provide a needed hour or two of relaxation, and the cancer patient will truly feel pampered.

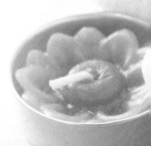

When someone calls with the question, "What can I do for you?", give them the name and phone number of your beauty salon, spa, or barber. Suggest surprising you with whatever tickles their fancy, and an hour or two of luxury would be just what the doctor prescribed. You will help your friend or family member just from making the suggestion, and just imagine how great you'll feel after the pampering!

When friends and family members are far away from a loved one diagnosed with cancer, and travel is out of the question or nearly impossible, plan to make a video or audio recording of greetings and send it to the patient. Ask relatives and buddies to record words of encouragement along with wishes for a full and speedy recovery. Sharing a recording of funny memories and old stories is a gift that will be enjoyed and remembered for many a year to come.

Can't visit friends and family due to your recent surgery? No problem—just put the recording they have sent you in your computer or television; wrap yourself in a cozy blanket; and heat up some hot apple cider and popcorn. Enjoy messages and greetings from those you love who are with you in spirit, if not "in the flesh."

"Whether we see them or not,

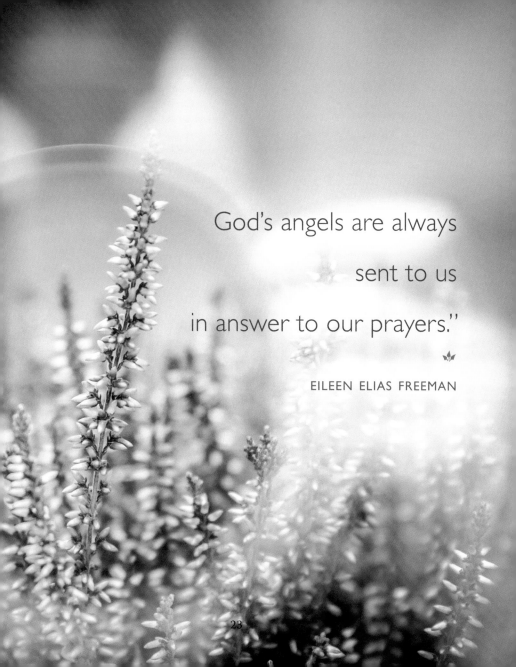

God's angels are always

sent to us

in answer to our prayers.''

EILEEN ELIAS FREEMAN

Six Down Six to Go

A Guide Through Chemotherapy

Any patient facing months, or perhaps years, of chemotherapy treatments needs lots of support and encouragement. This is the time to pull out all the stops, and to offer life-size gestures of kindness and caring. Usually by this point in the journey, the patient feels comfortable asking and receiving assistance.

"All the beautiful sentiments
in the world
weigh less than
a single lovely action."

🌿

JAMES RUSSELL LOWELL

With any season in full gear comes a variety of outdoor tasks that can seem overwhelming to someone facing cancer. Offer to rake and bag leaves, trim trees and bushes, or plant bulbs to bring delight in the spring. Washing windows or cleaning out gutters would be a fabulous way to help. Wash patio furniture and cushions and help put them away for the winter or get them out in the spring. Your friend or loved one will look around in delight when they know you've helped with the spring/summer/fall/winter cleanup!

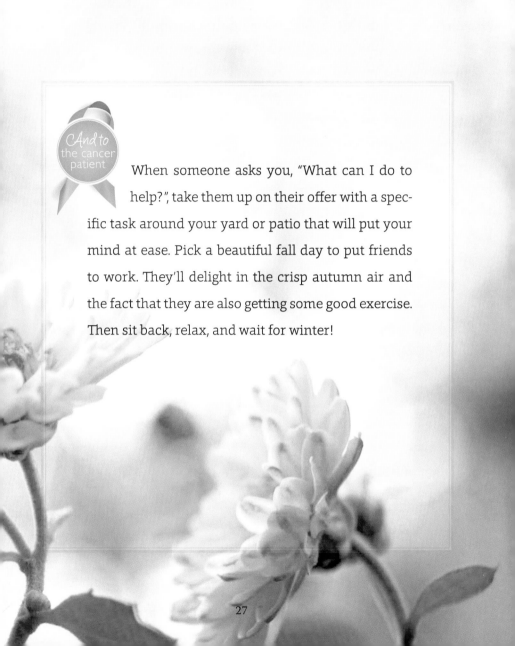

And to the cancer patient

When someone asks you, "What can I do to help?", take them up on their offer with a specific task around your yard or patio that will put your mind at ease. Pick a beautiful fall day to put friends to work. They'll delight in the crisp autumn air and the fact that they are also getting some good exercise. Then sit back, relax, and wait for winter!

$\mathcal{M}$usic can truly soothe any soul, so make arrangements to have a musician come to the cancer patient's home for an hour. If the patient has a piano, hire a pianist—amateur or professional. If not, a harpist, flutist, or even a harmonica player can bring an hour of relaxation and joy to any cancer patient. Contact your local colleges, churches, or even high schools to see if you can find a volunteer. Then make arrangements to join your friend or loved one for your own special concert. It will be an hour you will never forget!

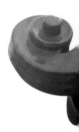

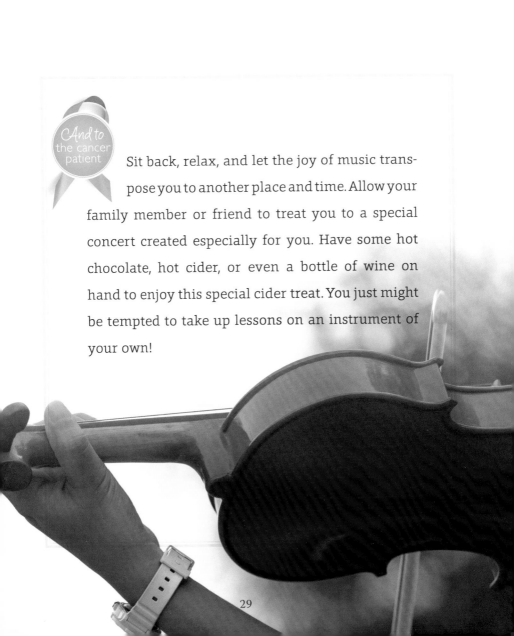

Sit back, relax, and let the joy of music transpose you to another place and time. Allow your family member or friend to treat you to a special concert created especially for you. Have some hot chocolate, hot cider, or even a bottle of wine on hand to enjoy this special cider treat. You just might be tempted to take up lessons on an instrument of your own!

"May you have a song in your heart

A smile on your lips

And nothing but joy at your fingertips."

AN IRISH BLESSING

A WALK
in the
PARK

It's so easy to get caught up in our own lives and forget about the friend or loved one who is facing their cancer every day. We mean well, but it's human nature to put off calling, writing, or even telling someone, "I love you." Let's all stop to smell the roses and even pick one or two along the way.

"From here to there,

from there to here,

funny things

are everywhere!"

DR. SEUSS

*S*tart a collection of something whimsical or comforting that can help your friend or loved one find something fun to focus on. If the patient is into pets, an array of stuffed, ceramic, glass, paper, or china bears, rabbits, cats, frogs, or pigs can become a friendly bedside support group. Marbles, quilts, and exquisite rocks for an outdoor garden can be given by all who come to visit. Soon the patient will have an accumulation of items that will remind them daily how much people care for them.

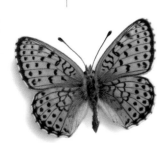
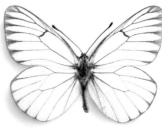
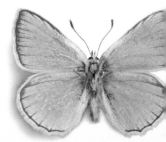

If you have always wanted to start a collection or already have the beginnings of one, spread the word that you hope to have the world's best collection of teacups, humor dvds, or birdhouses by the time you finish your treatments. Your friends and family will have a ball searching high and low for that very special "one," and it will give you something to concentrate on besides your treatments. Happy collecting!

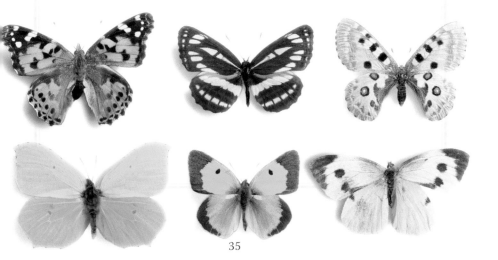

*P*eople going through cancer treatment often feel unattractive due to hair loss, weight changes, problems with their complexion, or just not feeling "up to par." It's amazing what a compliment can do to lift one's spirits! Look the cancer patient in the eye and tell them they look GREAT! Call attention to the positive changes or just the fact that the patient has made an effort to get out of the house to go to a movie or meet you for lunch. You'll be amazed at the positive reaction an encouraging word can bring. A smile on the face of a cancer patient will not only make their day… it will make yours, too.

When someone gives you a compliment while you're going through your treatments, take it as an acknowledgment that you really are doing a great job! It takes an effort to get up and face each day when you don't feel well or have lost the confidence in your appearance. Remember: the changes are usually temporary. One day soon, it will all be behind you.

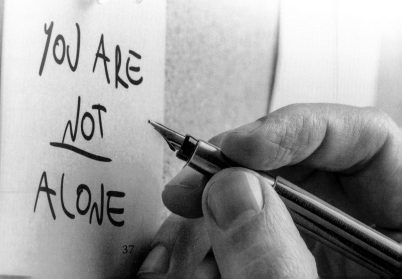

"In every man's heart
there is a secret nerve
that answers to
the vibrations of beauty."

CHRISTOPHER MORLEY

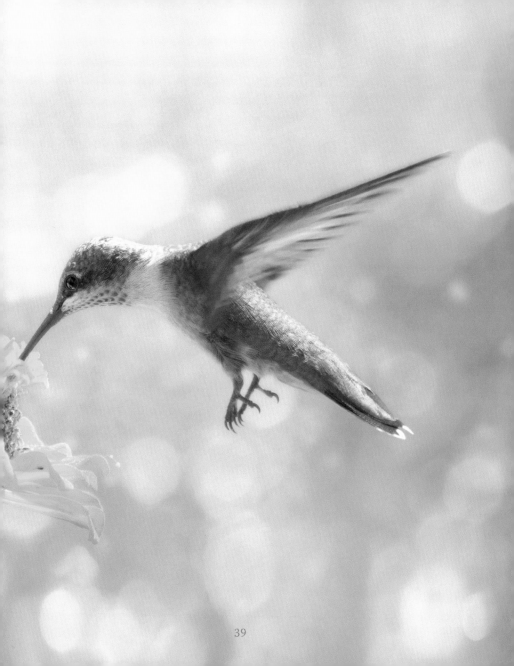

REAL SUPPORT
During Radiation Therapy

Statistics show that people facing cancer are more frightened about radiation therapy than any other form of treatment. In reality, it's not too bad at all— mostly a major inconvenience because it happens every day for usually several weeks. Support is needed now more than ever, as the number one side effect from radiation is exhaustion.

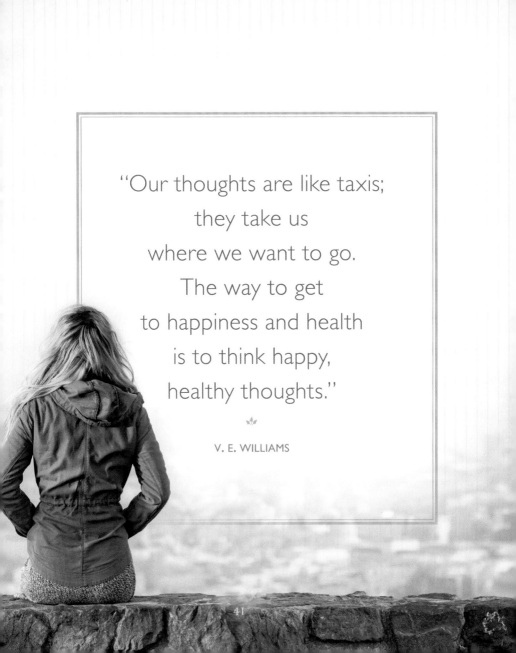

"Our thoughts are like taxis;
they take us
where we want to go.
The way to get
to happiness and health
is to think happy,
healthy thoughts."

V. E. WILLIAMS

*L*et's face it . . . we all hate car problems. But a mishap or breakdown; even routine maintenance can be overwhelming to someone going through radiation therapy. Offer to take the patient's car in for its annual checkup (oil change, fluid levels, tire pressure, etc.). Fill their car up with a full tank of gas. Get the car washed inside and out, perhaps adding a small cup of flowers in the beverage holder. If an accident has occurred, offer to get the estimates and schedule the appointment to get those dents removed. Your friend or loved one will be overwhelmed with your generous offer to help and may just use the time you've saved them to take that necessary nap.

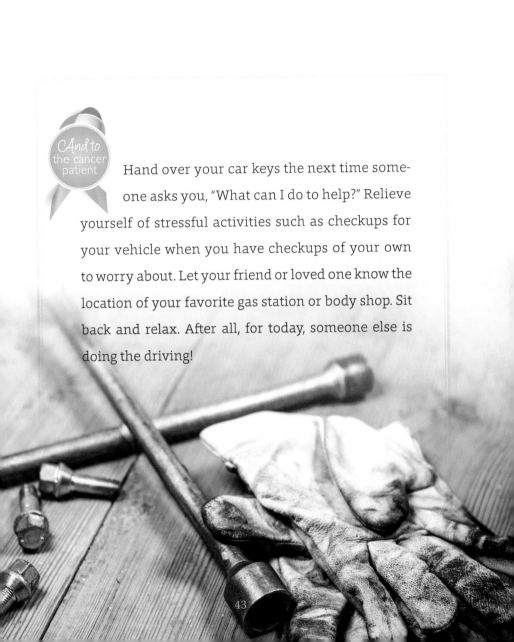

Hand over your car keys the next time someone asks you, "What can I do to help?" Relieve yourself of stressful activities such as checkups for your vehicle when you have checkups of your own to worry about. Let your friend or loved one know the location of your favorite gas station or body shop. Sit back and relax. After all, for today, someone else is doing the driving!

BACK INTO THE Mainstream of Life

One of the most important days in the life of every cancer patients is that infamous last day of treatment. Whether it's the final treatment of radiation therapy or the very last chemotherapy, the day is anticipated with a mixture of joy, accomplishment, relief, sadness, and fear.

"There's no thrill in easy sailing
When the skies are clear and blue,
There's no joy
in merely doing things
Which anyone can do.
But there is some satisfaction
That is mighty sweet to take,
When you reach a destination that
You thought you'd never make."

❧

SPIRELLA

*M*ark your calendar and make a point of contacting the cancer patient to congratulate them and wish them well. A call, card, or a bottle of champagne can go a long way towards telling your friend or loved one:

July

November

"You did it!"

And If
THE END IS NEAR...

Alas, even the strongest fighters may lose their battle against cancer. It's a tough disease, and providing support at the bitter end, if it comes, is the truest display of friendship. It's hard for us to see someone facing the end of their life, and it's human nature to want to remember someone "like they used to be." Don't desert your loved one or friend at this very critical time.

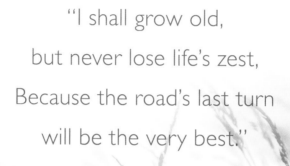

"I shall grow old,

but never lose life's zest,

Because the road's last turn

will be the very best."

HENRY VAN DYKE

*I*f a friend or loved one has been moved into hospice or is having home hospice care, do your very best to stop by more than once and pay your respects and love. It's easy to say, "I want to remember her as she was," but the end of life is a time when the cancer patient needs to feel loved and not forgotten. The patient may only be able to sit for a few minutes, and conversation may be difficult. But just resting your hand on theirs will let them know you were with them until the end.

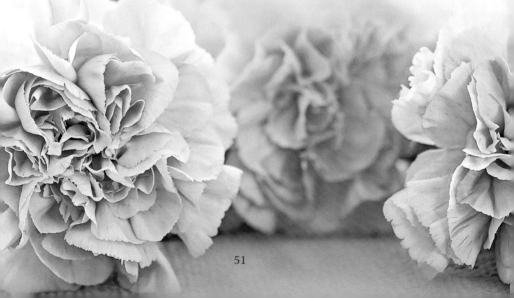

It may be difficult to swallow or speak, but when you are able, allow your family members and friends to pay their last respects. Just the comfort of their brief visit will remind you of the happy times you spent together and will remind you of the love you share with your visitor.

Celebration
OF LIFE:
We Did It!

The years pass by and with the love and support of family, friends, coworkers, employers, and total strangers, cancer survivors are living longer than ever before. Their lives will never be the same, but that doesn't mean that they can't have a wonderful new life—even a better life. Remember that your friend or loved one has been through an enormous challenge, and help them celebrate their grand accomplishment with continuous small acts of kindness and caring.

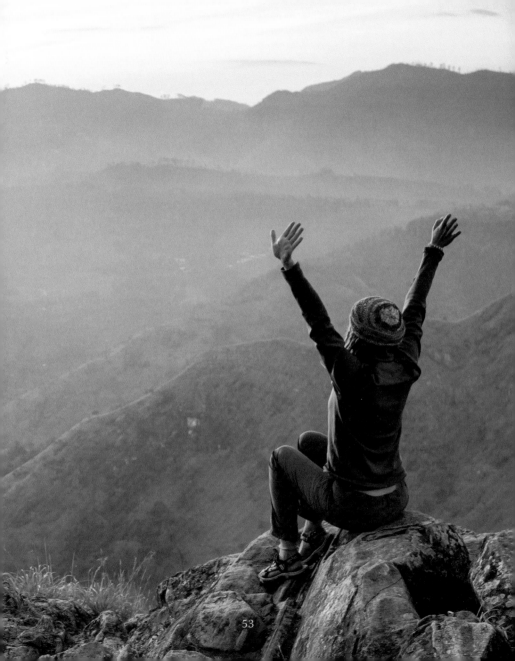

A real day brightener for any cancer patient is receiving mail—a note, a card, an article that lets them know you are thinking about them. Write a "Thank You" note to your friend or family member who has cancer that tells them how much you appreciate their friendship. Thank them for the different things they have done to bring joy and laughter into your life. Remind them of some little gesture they did that made your day. The patient will savor the memories and will most certainly feel loved and thought of for the rest of the day.

Design a simple "Thank You" note of your own
that you can return to friends and family members who do something special for you. Here's one
written by a special friend of The Cancer Club®:

For all your good wishes and candy
The balloons and stuffed animals were dandy.
Contributions, beautiful flowers, gourmet meals
And games—It's hard to keep track
        of all of the names.
Cards, books, visits, calls on the phone
Gave strength to me; I was never alone
Your hopes and prayers are appreciated
    more than I can say—
Hopes and dreams for a brighter day.
        MANY THANKS!!

How Can I Help?

© 2018 KPT Publishing, LLC
Written by Christine Clifford

Published by KPT Publishing
Minneapolis, Minnesota 55406
www.KPTPublishing.com

ISBN 978-1-944833-43-5

Designed by AbelerDesign.com

First printing March 2018

10 9 8 7 6 5 4 3 2 1

Printed in the United States of America

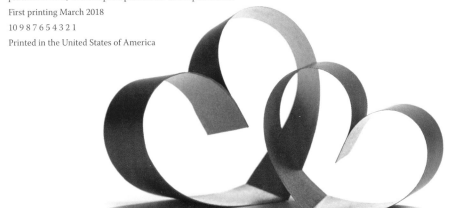

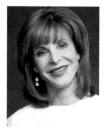

BEFORE HER FIRST BOUT with breast cancer, Christine Clifford had definitely cracked the glass ceiling. At the age of forty, she was senior vice president for the SPAR Group, an international information and merchandising services firm in New York.

Diagnosed with breast cancer in December 1994, she went on to write five humorous portrayals of her story in books entitled, *Now Now…I'm Having a No Hair Day!, Our Family Has Cancer, Too!* (written especially for children), *Cancer Has Its Privileges: Stories of Hope & Laughter, Laugh 'Til It Heals: Notes from the World's Funniest Cancer Mailbox,* and *Your Guardian Angel's Gift.*

Christine is currently president and chief executive officer of The Cancer Club®, a company designed to market humorous and helpful products for people with cancer. Now a two-time survivor, she speaks to organizations worldwide about finding humor and getting through life's adversities.

She lives with her husband, Dan, in both Florida and Minnesota and is a doting Grammy to her grandchildren, Katelyn and Kai.

Check out her websites at www.cancerclub.com and www.ChristineClifford.com

Don't forget to laugh!™

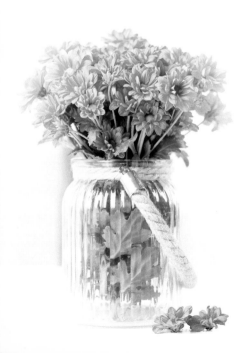

NOTES

NOTES

NOTES

NOTES